IRON DEFICIENCY ANEMIA

COOKBOOK

A Comprehensive Guide to Crafting Your Anemia-Fighting Diet

DR. ADAM MARTINEZ

Disclaimer

The information provided in this book is for educational and informational purposes only. It is not intended as a substitute for professional medical advice, diagnosis, or treatment. Always seek the advice of your physician or other qualified healthcare provider with any questions you may have regarding a medical condition or treatment.

The content of this book is based on general knowledge and research available up to the time of its publication. Health and medical information are subject to constant advancements and changes. Therefore, the author, publisher, and any contributors to this book make no representations or warranties of any kind, express or implied, regarding the accuracy, completeness,

suitability, or applicability of the
information contained herein.

Readers are encouraged to consult their
healthcare providers before making any
changes to their diet, exercise routines, or
medical treatment plans. Individual
responses to dietary and lifestyle changes
can vary, and what works for one person
may not work for another.

The author and publisher of this book are
not responsible for any adverse effects,
injuries, or damages arising from the
information provided within these pages.
Any reliance you place on the information in
this book is strictly at your own risk.
Please consult your healthcare provider
before beginning any new dietary or exercise

program, making changes to your existing treatment plan, or relying on the information presented in this book. Your healthcare provider is the best source of information regarding your individual health situation.

By reading and utilizing the information in this book, you agree to the terms of this disclaimer. If you do not agree with these terms, please refrain from using this book.

Remember that the field of health and medicine is complex and rapidly evolving. The information in this book is not a substitute for professional medical advice, and readers should always prioritize their health and safety by consulting qualified healthcare professionals.

Table of content

Introduction to Iron Deficiency Anemia   **7**

    Understanding Iron Deficiency Anemia   11

    Importance of Iron in the Diet   15

Building a Balanced Anemia-Fighting Diet   **21**

    Key Nutrients for Managing Anemia   26

    Planning Meals to Boost Iron Absorption   31

Iron-Rich Ingredients and Foods   **36**

    Lean Meats and Poultry   40

    Plant-Based Sources of Iron (Legumes, Grains, Nuts, Seeds)   45

    Dark Leafy Greens and Vegetables   50

    Fortified Foods and Supplements   55

Delicious Breakfast Recipes   **60**

    Spinach and Mushroom Omelette   64

    Iron-Boosting Smoothie Bowl   67

    Quinoa Breakfast Porridge   70

Nutrient-Packed Lunch Ideas   **73**

    Lentil and Chickpea Salad   77

    Turkey and Spinach Wrap   81

    Tofu and Vegetable Stir-Fry   85

Wholesome Dinner Dishes   **89**

    Beef and Broccoli Stir-Fry   93

    Salmon with Quinoa and Asparagus   98

    Black Bean and Sweet Potato Chili   101

Snacks and Sides for Sustained Energy   **105**

    Roasted Chickpea Snack   109

    Hummus and Veggie Platter   112

    Iron-Rich Trail Mix   116

Sweet Treats for Anemia Support   **118**

    Dark Chocolate Nut Bites   122

    Berry and Spinach Smoothie   126

    Iron-Enriched Dessert Options   129

Lifestyle Tips to Enhance Iron Absorption   **133**

    Pairing Foods for Better Iron Uptake   138

    Cooking Techniques to Preserve Iron Content   142

    Managing Iron Intake with Other Nutrients   146

Meal Planning and Grocery Shopping for Anemia **151**

    Weekly Meal Plans   156

    Stocking Your Pantry with Iron-Rich Foods   161

    Reading Labels and Choosing Fortified Products 166

Frequently Asked Questions about Anemia and Diet 170

    Addressing Concerns About Vegetarian or Vegan
Diets   176

Conclusion and Empowerment   **181**

Introduction to Iron Deficiency Anemia

Welcome to a world where an unassuming mineral, iron, holds the key to a vibrant life. Imagine this element as a superhero, silently working behind the scenes to keep you strong and full of energy. As we journey through this introduction, you'll uncover the secret role iron plays in your body, how its absence can lead to tiredness and weakness, and most importantly, how you can harness its power to regain your vitality.

Now, let's meet Sam, a person just like you. One day, while scrolling through his Facebook feed, he stumbled upon a shared link to the "Iron Deficiency Anemia Cookbook." Intrigued, he clicked the link, and a world of knowledge opened up before him.

Sam's story is like yours - he had been feeling tired and drained, thinking it was just part of life's ups and downs. But as he read the stories of real people who faced similar struggles, a spark ignited within him. He realized he didn't have to accept feeling this way; there was hope.

The cookbook revealed simple yet powerful ways to fight back against fatigue. Sam learned about iron-rich foods and how they could infuse his body with renewed energy. Spinach, lean meats, and other delicious options became his allies in this journey to reclaim his vitality.

As weeks passed, Sam's transformation was undeniable. His friends noticed his healthier glow and his newfound zest for life. Sam shared his story on Facebook, and his friends, inspired by his journey, joined him in exploring the world of iron-rich foods.

Dear reader, you hold the key to your own vitality within these pages. Just as Sam's life changed, so too can yours. Let the wisdom within this cookbook be your guide to a stronger, more vibrant you. The journey starts now – embrace the power of iron and unlock the energy that's been waiting for you.

Are you ready to embark on your journey towards renewed vitality? Turn the page and discover the transformative potential of the

"Iron Deficiency Anemia Cookbook." Join Sam and countless others in reclaiming your energy and embracing a life of strength and well-being. Your adventure awaits!

Understanding Iron Deficiency Anemia

At times, our bodies wage silent battles that affect our vitality more than we realize. Iron deficiency anemia is one such battle – a condition that stealthily chips away at our energy, leaving us weary and drained. In this chapter, we will unravel the mystery behind this common yet often misunderstood adversary.

Picture your bloodstream as a bustling highway, with oxygen-carrying red blood cells as the vehicles. Iron plays a crucial role in producing these vehicles, ensuring they can efficiently transport oxygen to every corner of your body. Now imagine what happens when there's not enough iron – the highway becomes congested, and your body's energy production grinds to a halt.

In these pages, we will delve into the mechanics of iron deficiency anemia. We'll demystify medical terms, helping you understand the signs and symptoms that may be lurking in the shadows. From the pale hue that can drape your skin to the weariness that seeps into your bones, we'll connect the dots between these everyday experiences and the underlying battle for iron.

But don't worry, we won't leave you in the dark. Armed with knowledge, you'll be empowered to recognize the subtle signals your body sends. You'll learn about the risk factors that can tip the scales toward anemia, such as certain diets, medical conditions, or even life stages.

By the time you reach the end of this chapter, you'll see iron deficiency anemia for what it truly is – a foe that can be understood and, most importantly, conquered. With every turn of the page, you'll gather the insights needed to emerge victorious in this battle for boundless energy and well-being.

So, dear reader, let's embark on this enlightening journey together. Arm yourself with understanding and prepare to unveil the hidden battle within – the battle against iron deficiency anemia. Your knowledge will be your shield, and your determination your sword. Onward, to grasp the reins of your vitality once more!

Importance of Iron in the Diet

Iron is an essential mineral that plays a pivotal role in maintaining human health and well-being. It is a vital component of various physiological processes within the body, ranging from oxygen transport to energy production. While the importance of iron in the diet is widely acknowledged, its significance often goes beyond its basic functions, extending to the prevention of various health conditions and the promotion of overall vitality.

Oxygen Transport and Hemoglobin Formation:

One of the most crucial roles of iron is its involvement in the production of hemoglobin, a protein found in red blood cells that carries oxygen from the lungs to different parts of the body. Without adequate iron intake, the body cannot produce sufficient hemoglobin, leading to anemia – a condition characterized by fatigue, weakness, and reduced physical endurance. Including iron-rich foods in the diet ensures proper oxygen transport, thereby supporting optimal bodily functions.

Energy Production:

Iron is a key component of enzymes involved in the energy production process. These enzymes are responsible for converting nutrients into energy that the body can utilize for various activities. A deficiency in iron can lead to reduced energy levels, making individuals more prone to fatigue and lethargy. By incorporating iron-rich foods into their diets, individuals can help maintain consistent energy levels throughout the day.

Cognitive Function and Brain Health:
Iron plays a significant role in maintaining cognitive function and brain health. It supports the synthesis of neurotransmitters, such as dopamine and serotonin, which are essential for mood regulation, stress management, and overall mental well-being. Inadequate iron intake has been linked to impaired cognitive performance, decreased attention span, and an increased risk of neurodevelopmental disorders.

Immune System Support:

Iron contributes to a robust immune system by aiding in the production of immune cells and antibodies that defend the body against infections and diseases. A well-functioning immune system is crucial for preventing illnesses and promoting overall health. Including iron-rich foods in the diet can help strengthen the body's defense mechanisms.

Growth and Development:

Iron is particularly important during periods of rapid growth and development, such as infancy, childhood, and adolescence. It supports the formation of new cells, tissues, and muscles, and contributes to overall growth and maturation. A deficiency in iron during these critical stages can lead to developmental delays and growth impairments.

Importance for Specific Groups:

Certain groups of people, such as pregnant women, athletes, and vegetarians, have increased iron requirements due to factors like higher blood volume, increased physical activity, and reduced iron absorption from plant-based sources. Adequate iron intake is especially important for these individuals to meet their unique nutritional needs and maintain optimal health.

Incorporating iron-rich foods into the diet is essential for maintaining good health and preventing a range of potential health issues. From supporting oxygen transport and energy production to promoting cognitive function and immune system support, iron's multifaceted role underscores its significance in overall well-being. Educating individuals about the importance of iron and encouraging them to make conscious dietary choices can contribute to a healthier, more vibrant life.

Building a Balanced Anemia-Fighting Diet

In a world where fast-paced lives often dictate our choices, it's easy to overlook the silent epidemic that can sap our vitality: anemia. This common condition, characterized by a deficiency of red blood cells or hemoglobin, can lead to fatigue, weakness, and a lack of energy. However, armed with the right knowledge and a balanced approach to nutrition, you can take charge of your well-being and construct an anemia-fighting diet that empowers your health from within. By incorporating a variety of nutrient-rich foods, you can combat anemia and pave the way for a vibrant, energetic life.

The Foundation: Iron-Rich Foods:

At the heart of any anemia-fighting diet lies a robust intake of iron-rich foods. Iron is the building block of hemoglobin, the molecule that transports oxygen throughout your body. Opt for lean meats such as poultry, fish, and lean cuts of beef to infuse your diet with heme iron - a form of iron that is readily absorbed by the body. For vegetarians and vegans, plant-based sources like beans, lentils, tofu, and spinach provide non-heme iron, which, when combined with vitamin C-rich foods like citrus fruits and bell peppers, enhances iron absorption.

Fueling with Folate and Vitamin B12:

Equally essential to combatting anemia are folate and vitamin B12. These B-vitamins play a pivotal role in the formation of red blood cells and DNA synthesis. Incorporate a variety of leafy greens, fortified cereals, and legumes to amp up your folate intake. To ensure sufficient vitamin B12, embrace dairy products, eggs, and fortified plant-based alternatives. These nutrients work in tandem to support red blood cell production and fortify your body's defense against anemia.

Enriching with Vitamin C and Copper: The road to anemia prevention is paved with synergistic partnerships between key nutrients. Vitamin C, often celebrated for its immune-boosting properties, also aids in the absorption of non-heme iron. Citrus fruits, strawberries, and broccoli serve as delightful additions to your diet, enhancing the iron-absorption potential of plant-based foods. Copper, too, deserves a spotlight for its role in iron metabolism. Nuts, seeds, whole grains, and shellfish introduce this trace mineral to your plate, contributing to a well-rounded anemia-fighting strategy.

Balancing with a Rainbow of Nutrients:

A diverse and colorful array of fruits and vegetables not only elevates your diet's visual appeal but also delivers a symphony of nutrients crucial for anemia prevention. Vitamin A, found in vibrant orange and dark leafy green vegetables, promotes healthy red blood cell production. Zinc, abundant in lean meats, dairy, and legumes, supports immune function and assists in iron utilization. Incorporating a rainbow of nutrient-dense foods not only fuels your body with vitality but also bolsters its defenses against anemia's grip.

Building a balanced anemia-fighting diet is a transformative journey toward renewed energy and vitality. By carefully selecting iron-rich foods, harnessing the power of B-vitamins, embracing vitamin C and copper, and infusing your diet with a diverse array of nutrients, you are forging a path toward optimal health. Empower yourself with the knowledge that you hold the key to fortifying your body against anemia's challenges. Through mindful dietary choices, you can paint a vibrant canvas of well-being, ensuring that each meal becomes a step toward a life brimming with energy and vitality.

Key Nutrients for Managing Anemia

Managing anemia requires a strategic focus on key nutrients that play a vital role in combating this condition. Here are the essential nutrients to prioritize:

- Iron: A cornerstone in anemia management, iron is crucial for the production of hemoglobin, which carries oxygen to your body's cells. Include both heme iron (from animal sources like lean meats) and non-heme iron (from plant-based sources like beans, lentils, and spinach) to ensure optimal iron intake.

- Vitamin B12: This vitamin is essential for red blood cell formation and neurological health. Incorporate foods like lean meats, fish, dairy, eggs, and fortified plant-based alternatives to maintain adequate vitamin B12 levels.

- Folate (Vitamin B9): Vital for DNA synthesis and cell division, folate is pivotal in preventing anemia. Leafy greens, fortified cereals, legumes, and citrus fruits are excellent sources of this nutrient.

- Vitamin C: Enhances the absorption of non-heme iron from plant-based sources. Include citrus fruits, strawberries, bell peppers, and broccoli to improve iron uptake.

- Copper: Supports iron metabolism and aids in the formation of hemoglobin. Nuts, seeds, whole grains, and shellfish are rich sources of copper.

- Vitamin A: Essential for healthy red blood cell production and maintaining proper immune function. Carrots, sweet potatoes, dark leafy greens, and bell peppers are rich in vitamin A.
- Zinc: Assists in iron utilization and supports immune function. Include lean meats, dairy products, legumes, and whole grains to ensure sufficient zinc intake.
- Vitamin E: Offers antioxidant protection to red blood cells and supports overall cellular health. Nuts, seeds, and vegetable oils are good sources of vitamin E.

- Vitamin K: Important for blood clotting and bone health. Leafy greens, broccoli, and Brussels sprouts are high in vitamin K.

- B Vitamins (B6, B2, B3): These vitamins contribute to red blood cell production and energy metabolism. Incorporate a variety of whole grains, lean meats, nuts, and dairy products to meet your B-vitamin needs.

- Protein: Adequate protein intake is essential for the production of hemoglobin and overall cell health. Include lean meats, poultry, fish, dairy, legumes, and plant-based protein sources.

Remember, a balanced diet that includes a variety of nutrient-rich foods is key to managing anemia effectively. Consult with a healthcare professional or registered dietitian for personalized guidance based on your specific nutritional needs and health status.

Planning Meals to Boost Iron Absorption

Boosting iron absorption through meal planning involves strategic pairing of iron-rich foods with enhancers like vitamin C and avoiding inhibitors that hinder absorption. Here's a guide to help you plan meals that maximize iron uptake:

- Iron-Rich Foods: Incorporate good sources of heme and non-heme iron into your meals. Heme iron is found in animal products like lean meats (chicken, turkey, lean beef) and fish (salmon, tuna). Non-heme iron is abundant in plant-based foods such as beans, lentils, tofu, spinach, and fortified cereals.

- Vitamin C Enhancers: Include vitamin C-rich foods in your meals to enhance non-heme iron absorption. Citrus fruits (oranges, grapefruits), strawberries, bell peppers, broccoli, and kiwi are excellent options. Add these fruits or vegetables to your iron-rich dishes or enjoy them as snacks.
- Iron-Fortified Foods: Opt for iron-fortified foods like cereals and plant-based milk alternatives (soy, almond, oat) to increase your iron intake.
- Pairing Ideas: Create powerful iron-absorption combinations, such as:

a. Spinach salad with grilled chicken, strawberries, and citrus vinaigrette.

b. Lentil soup with a side of bell pepper and orange slices.

c. Tofu stir-fry with broccoli, bell peppers, and brown rice.

d. Oatmeal topped with fortified almond milk, sliced almonds, and mixed berries.

- Limit Inhibitors: Some foods can hinder iron absorption. Reduce consumption of calcium-rich foods (dairy) and tannin-containing beverages (tea, coffee) during iron-rich meals. Also, avoid consuming high-fiber foods (whole grains, bran) and phytates-rich foods (whole grains, legumes) in excess with iron-rich meals.

- Cooking Techniques: Certain cooking methods can enhance iron absorption. Consider using cast iron cookware for preparing iron-rich foods. Cooking foods like tomatoes with iron-rich ingredients can increase iron uptake.

- Small, Frequent Meals: Distribute iron-rich foods and enhancers across multiple meals and snacks throughout the day for consistent iron absorption.

- Hydration: Stay adequately hydrated, as fluids support digestion and nutrient absorption.

- Supplements: If recommended by a healthcare professional, take iron supplements with vitamin C-rich foods to enhance absorption.

However, consult a healthcare provider before starting any supplementation.

- Consult a Professional: For personalized guidance, consult a registered dietitian or healthcare provider, especially if you have specific dietary needs or health conditions.

Remember, balance is key. Aim for a variety of nutrient-rich foods in your diet to support overall health while strategically optimizing iron absorption for effective anemia management.

Iron-Rich Ingredients and Foods

Incorporating iron-rich ingredients and foods into your diet is essential for maintaining healthy iron levels and preventing anemia. Here's a list of iron-rich options to consider:

Heme Iron Sources (Animal-Based):
- Lean red meats (beef, lamb)
- Poultry (chicken, turkey)
- Fish (salmon, tuna, sardines)
- Organ meats (liver)
- Shellfish (oysters, clams, mussels)
- Eggs (especially egg yolks)

Non-Heme Iron Sources (Plant-Based):
- Legumes (beans, lentils, chickpeas)
- Tofu and tempeh

- Nuts and seeds (pumpkin seeds, sesame seeds)
- Fortified cereals and whole grains (quinoa, oatmeal)
- Spinach and other leafy greens (kale, collard greens)
- Broccoli and Brussels sprouts
- Dried fruits (apricots, raisins)
- Molasses

Combining Iron-Rich Foods with Enhancers:

- Pair non-heme iron sources with vitamin C-rich foods to enhance absorption. Examples include adding bell peppers, citrus fruits, strawberries, or tomatoes to iron-rich meals.
- Consume iron-fortified foods, like cereals and plant-based milk

alternatives, which often contain added iron and nutrients.

Cooking Tips to Maximize Iron Absorption:

- Use cast iron cookware for preparing iron-rich foods.

- Cook foods like tomatoes with iron-containing ingredients to boost absorption.

- Avoid excessive consumption of calcium-rich foods (dairy) or tannin-containing beverages (tea, coffee) during iron-rich meals, as they can hinder absorption.

Sample Iron-Rich Meals:

- Grilled chicken salad with spinach, bell peppers, strawberries, and citrus vinaigrette.

- Lentil stew with tomatoes, broccoli, and a slice of whole-grain bread.
- Tofu stir-fry with mixed vegetables and quinoa.
- Oatmeal topped with pumpkin seeds, dried apricots, and fortified almond milk.

Remember, balance is key. While incorporating iron-rich foods, also aim for a varied and nutrient-rich diet that includes other essential vitamins and minerals to support overall health. If you have specific dietary needs or health conditions, consider consulting a registered dietitian for personalized guidance.

Lean Meats and Poultry

Lean meats and poultry are excellent sources of high-quality protein, essential nutrients, and, in the case of lean meats, heme iron. Incorporating lean cuts of these meats into your diet can provide numerous health benefits. Here's a closer look at lean meats and poultry:

Lean Meats:

Lean meats refer to cuts of meat that have lower fat content compared to fattier cuts. They are rich in protein, vitamins, and minerals, making them a valuable addition to a balanced diet. Some examples of lean meats include:

- Skinless Chicken Breast: A versatile and widely enjoyed option that is low in fat and high in protein.
- Turkey Breast: Similar to chicken breast, turkey is lean and packed with protein.
- Lean Beef Cuts: Cuts such as sirloin, tenderloin, and eye of round are lean options that provide protein and heme iron.
- Pork Tenderloin: A lean cut of pork that is tender and flavorful.

Nutritional Benefits:
- Protein: Lean meats are rich sources of high-quality protein, essential for muscle growth, repair, and overall body function.
- Iron: Lean meats, especially red meats, provide heme iron, which is

easily absorbed by the body and important for oxygen transport.

- B Vitamins: These meats contain B vitamins like B12, which is crucial for nerve function and DNA synthesis.
- Zinc: An essential mineral that supports immune function, wound healing, and metabolism.

Cooking Tips:

- Trim visible fat before cooking to reduce overall fat content.
- Use healthy cooking methods like grilling, baking, broiling, or steaming to retain nutrients without adding excess fats.
- Avoid breading or frying, as these methods can increase calorie and fat content.

Balanced Diet:

- While lean meats offer valuable nutrients, it's important to maintain a balanced diet that includes a variety of protein sources, such as plant-based proteins (beans, lentils, tofu) and seafood. Incorporate plenty of fruits, vegetables, whole grains, and other nutrient-rich foods for optimal health.

Individual Considerations:

If you have dietary restrictions, health conditions, or ethical preferences, consult a registered dietitian or healthcare professional to tailor your diet accordingly.

Remember, moderation and variety are key. Lean meats and poultry can be part of a healthful diet, but it's important to incorporate a wide range of nutrient sources to meet your overall nutritional needs.

Plant-Based Sources of Iron (Legumes, Grains, Nuts, Seeds)

Plant-based sources of iron are an essential part of a balanced diet, especially for those following a vegetarian or vegan lifestyle. These foods are rich in non-heme iron, which is not as easily absorbed as heme iron from animal sources but can still contribute significantly to your iron intake. Here are some plant-based sources of iron from legumes, grains, nuts, and seeds:

Legumes:

- Beans (Black beans, kidney beans, chickpeas, lentils, etc.): These are versatile and protein-packed sources of iron, perfect for soups, stews, salads, and more.

- Tofu and Tempeh: Soy-based products like tofu and tempeh are not only rich in iron but also provide a good amount of protein.
- Peas: Both green peas and split peas offer iron along with dietary fiber.

Grains:

- Quinoa: A nutrient-dense grain that contains a decent amount of iron and complete protein.
- Oats: Oats are not only a great source of fiber but also provide iron.
- Brown Rice: Whole grains like brown rice contribute iron to your diet.
- Fortified Cereals: Some cereals are fortified with iron and other nutrients, making them a convenient option.

Nuts and Seeds:

- Pumpkin Seeds: Also known as pepitas, these seeds are a good source of iron, zinc, and healthy fats.

- Sunflower Seeds: These crunchy seeds offer iron, vitamin E, and other nutrients.

- Sesame Seeds: These tiny seeds can be sprinkled on dishes for added iron and flavor.

- Cashews and Almonds: Nuts like cashews and almonds provide a dose of iron along with healthy fats.

Combining with Vitamin C-Rich Foods:

To enhance the absorption of non-heme iron from plant-based sources, pair them with foods high in vitamin C. For example, adding bell peppers, citrus fruits, strawberries, or tomatoes to your meals can increase iron uptake.

Cooking Tips:

- Soaking legumes before cooking can improve nutrient absorption and reduce cooking time.
- Cooking foods like tomatoes with iron-containing ingredients can boost absorption.
- If you're consuming plant-based iron sources alongside calcium-rich foods, consider separating them by a few hours to avoid inhibiting iron absorption.

Variety is Key:

It's important to include a variety of these plant-based sources of iron in your diet to ensure you're getting a well-rounded intake of nutrients. If you have specific dietary restrictions, health conditions, or concerns, consulting a registered dietitian can help you create a balanced and iron-rich plant-based diet that meets your individual needs.

Dark Leafy Greens and Vegetables

Dark leafy greens and vegetables are nutritional powerhouses, rich in vitamins, minerals, and antioxidants. Incorporating these nutrient-dense foods into your diet can provide numerous health benefits. Here are some examples of dark leafy greens and vegetables:

Dark Leafy Greens:

- Spinach: A versatile green that's packed with iron, folate, and vitamins A and K.
- Kale: A superfood rich in iron, calcium, vitamin K, and antioxidants.
- Swiss Chard: Contains iron, magnesium, potassium, and vitamins A and C.

- Collard Greens: A great source of calcium, vitamin K, and fiber.
- Mustard Greens: Provide iron, calcium, and vitamins A, C, and K.

Other Nutrient-Rich Vegetables:
- Broccoli: Rich in vitamin C, vitamin K, fiber, and various antioxidants.
- Brussels Sprouts: Packed with vitamin K, vitamin C, and fiber.
- Green Peas: Provide iron, protein, and dietary fiber.
- Asparagus: A source of folate, vitamin K, and antioxidants.
- Zucchini: Low in calories and rich in vitamin C and potassium.
- Green Beans: Contain iron, fiber, and vitamins A and C.

Benefits of Dark Leafy Greens and Vegetables:

- Nutrient Density: These foods offer a wide range of vitamins (A, C, K), minerals (iron, calcium, magnesium), and antioxidants, contributing to overall health.
- Iron Content: While the iron in plant-based sources is non-heme iron (less easily absorbed), pairing these foods with vitamin C-rich options can enhance iron absorption.
- Bone Health: Dark leafy greens are excellent sources of vitamin K and calcium, supporting bone health.
- Heart Health: Vegetables like broccoli and Brussels sprouts are associated with heart-protective effects due to their fiber and antioxidant content.

- Digestive Health: Fiber in these vegetables supports healthy digestion and gut function.

Incorporating Dark Leafy Greens and Vegetables:

- Salads: Create nutrient-packed salads with a variety of greens and colorful vegetables.

- Smoothies: Blend dark leafy greens into smoothies with fruits and a source of protein.

- Stir-Fries: Add vegetables like broccoli, bell peppers, and spinach to stir-fries and noodle dishes.

- Sides: Steam or roast vegetables as a delicious and nutritious side dish.

- Soups and Stews: Enhance the nutritional profile of soups and stews by adding greens like kale or spinach.

Remember, variety is key to a balanced diet. Incorporate a mix of different dark leafy greens and vegetables to ensure you're reaping the full spectrum of health benefits they offer. If you have dietary considerations or specific health goals, consulting a registered dietitian can help you create a personalized plan.

Fortified Foods and Supplements

Fortified foods and supplements can play a crucial role in meeting your nutritional needs, especially when it comes to specific nutrients that may be lacking in your diet. Here's a closer look at fortified foods and supplements:

Fortified Foods:

Fortified foods are products that have had specific nutrients added to them to enhance their nutritional content. Common nutrients that are added to fortified foods include vitamins (such as vitamin D, B vitamins, and folic acid) and minerals (such as iron and calcium). Examples of fortified foods include:

- Fortified Plant-Based Milks: Almond milk, soy milk, and oat milk are often fortified with calcium, vitamin D, and vitamin B12.
- Fortified Breakfast Cereals: Many breakfast cereals are fortified with vitamins and minerals like iron, folic acid, and B vitamins.
- Fortified Grains: Some types of rice, pasta, and bread are enriched with nutrients like iron and B vitamins.
- Fortified Nutritional Yeast: Often used by vegans as a cheese substitute, nutritional yeast is fortified with vitamin B12.
- Fortified Fruit Juices: Certain fruit juices are fortified with nutrients like calcium and vitamin D.

Supplements:

Supplements are concentrated sources of specific nutrients that can be taken in addition to your regular diet. They are often recommended to address deficiencies or specific health conditions. Some common supplements include:

- Multivitamins: These contain a combination of vitamins and minerals, offering a comprehensive approach to filling potential nutritional gaps.

- Single Nutrient Supplements: These provide a specific nutrient, such as iron, vitamin D, or omega-3 fatty acids, to target a particular deficiency or health concern.

- Plant-Based Supplements: Some supplements are designed specifically for those following vegetarian or vegan diets and may include nutrients like vitamin B12, iron, and omega-3s.

- Individualized Supplements: Based on medical advice, individuals may be prescribed supplements to address specific health conditions or deficiencies.

Considerations:

- Consult a Healthcare Professional: Before starting any supplements, it's important to consult with a healthcare provider or registered dietitian. They can help you determine if supplements are necessary and guide you on proper dosage.
- Food First: Whenever possible, try to obtain nutrients from whole foods. Fortified foods and supplements

should be used to complement a balanced diet, not replace it.

- Quality Matters: Choose reputable brands when selecting supplements, and be cautious of excessive dosages. Some nutrients can have adverse effects when taken in excess.

Personalization is Key:

Your nutritional needs are unique, and the decision to use fortified foods or supplements should be based on your individual dietary choices, health goals, and any specific deficiencies you may have. Working with a healthcare provider or registered dietitian can help you make informed choices that best support your well-being.

Delicious Breakfast Recipes

it's important to focus on incorporating iron-rich ingredients and pairing them with vitamin C sources to enhance absorption. Here are a couple of breakfast recipes that can help support your iron levels:

1. Iron-Boosting Breakfast Bowl:

Ingredients:

- 1/2 cup cooked quinoa (a good source of non-heme iron)
- 1/4 cup chopped dried apricots (source of iron)
- 1/4 cup sliced strawberries (vitamin C source)
- 1 tablespoon pumpkin seeds (source of iron and zinc)

- 1 tablespoon chopped almonds (source of iron)
- Greek yogurt or plant-based yogurt

Instructions:

- In a bowl, layer cooked quinoa.
- Top with chopped dried apricots, sliced strawberries, pumpkin seeds, and chopped almonds.
- Serve with a dollop of Greek yogurt or your favorite plant-based yogurt.

2. Spinach and Red Bell Pepper Omelette:

Ingredients:

- 2 eggs (or tofu for a vegan option)
- 1/2 cup chopped spinach (iron source)
- 1/4 cup diced red bell pepper (vitamin C source)
- Salt, pepper, and your favorite herbs/spices

- Olive oil or cooking spray

Instructions:

- In a bowl, whisk eggs (or crumbled tofu) with salt, pepper, and your choice of herbs/spices.
- In a non-stick pan, sauté diced red bell pepper until slightly softened.
- Add chopped spinach and cook until wilted.
- Push the veggies to one side of the pan and pour the egg mixture into the other side.
- Once the eggs are cooked, fold the omelette over the veggies.

Serve with a side of whole-grain toast.

These recipes focus on incorporating iron-rich ingredients like quinoa, spinach, dried apricots, and nuts, while also including vitamin C sources like strawberries and red bell pepper to enhance iron absorption. Remember to consult a healthcare professional or registered dietitian if you have specific dietary needs or concerns related to your iron deficiency anemia.

Spinach and Mushroom Omelette

Here's a recipe that combines these iron-rich ingredients while providing a delicious and nutritious meal:

Spinach and Mushroom Iron-Boosting Omelette:

Ingredients:

- 2 eggs (or tofu for a vegan option)
- 1/2 cup chopped spinach (iron source)
- 1/2 cup sliced mushrooms
- 1/4 cup diced onion
- 1/4 cup diced red bell pepper (vitamin C source)
- Salt, pepper, and your favorite herbs/spices
- Olive oil or cooking spray

Instructions:

- In a bowl, whisk eggs (or crumbled tofu) with a pinch of salt, pepper, and your choice of herbs/spices.
- In a non-stick pan, sauté diced onion until translucent.
- Add sliced mushrooms and cook until they release their moisture and start to brown.
- Push the mushrooms and onion to one side of the pan and add chopped spinach to the other side. Cook until wilted.
- Spread the veggies evenly in the pan and pour the egg mixture over them.
- Let the eggs set for a minute, then gently lift the edges and tilt the pan to allow the uncooked egg to flow underneath.

- Once the omelette is mostly set but still slightly runny on top, carefully fold it in half using a spatula.
- Continue cooking for another minute or until the eggs are fully cooked.
- Slide the omelette onto a plate, and top with diced red bell pepper.

Serve with a slice of whole-grain toast for an extra boost of fiber and nutrients.

This omelette combines iron-rich spinach and mushrooms with vitamin C from red bell pepper to help enhance iron absorption. It's a well-rounded and satisfying breakfast option for those dealing with iron deficiency anemia. As always, consult a healthcare professional or registered dietitian if you have specific dietary concerns or questions about managing your anemia.

Iron-Boosting Smoothie Bowl

Here's a delicious and nutritious iron-boosting smoothie bowl recipe that incorporates iron-rich ingredients and vitamin C to enhance iron absorption:

Iron-Boosting Smoothie Bowl:

Ingredients:

- 1 frozen banana
- 1/2 cup frozen mixed berries (blueberries, strawberries, raspberries)
- 1 cup fresh spinach (iron source)
- 1/2 cup plain Greek yogurt (or plant-based yogurt)
- 1 tablespoon chia seeds (source of iron)

- 1/2 cup orange juice (vitamin C source)
- Optional toppings: sliced kiwi, pumpkin seeds, almonds

Instructions:

- In a blender, combine the frozen banana, frozen mixed berries, fresh spinach, Greek yogurt, chia seeds, and orange juice.
- Blend until smooth and creamy. You can adjust the consistency by adding more orange juice if needed.
- Pour the smoothie into a bowl.
- Top with sliced kiwi, pumpkin seeds, and almonds for an extra boost of nutrients and crunch.
- Enjoy with a spoon!

This smoothie bowl is not only refreshing but also packed with iron from spinach and chia seeds, while the vitamin C-rich orange juice and berries help enhance iron absorption. It's a vibrant and satisfying breakfast option that can help support your iron deficiency anemia. Remember to consult a healthcare professional or registered dietitian if you have specific dietary needs or concerns.

Quinoa Breakfast Porridge

Here's a simple and delicious recipe for a quinoa breakfast porridge:

Iron-Boosting Quinoa Breakfast Porridge:

Ingredients:

- 1/2 cup quinoa, rinsed
- 1 cup water or milk of your choice (almond milk, soy milk, etc.)
- 1/2 teaspoon cinnamon
- 1/4 teaspoon vanilla extract
- 1 tablespoon chopped dried apricots (iron source)
- 1 tablespoon chopped almonds (iron source)
- 1/4 cup mixed berries (vitamin C source)

- Optional sweetener: honey, maple syrup, or stevia

Instructions:

- In a small saucepan, combine quinoa, water or milk, cinnamon, and vanilla extract.

- Bring to a boil, then reduce the heat to a simmer. Cover and cook for about 15-20 minutes, or until the quinoa is cooked and has absorbed the liquid. Stir occasionally.

- Once the quinoa is cooked, remove from heat and let it sit for a few minutes to thicken.

- Stir in the chopped dried apricots and chopped almonds.

- Transfer the quinoa porridge to a bowl.

- Top with mixed berries for a burst of vitamin C and added flavor.

- Drizzle with your preferred sweetener, if desired.

- Give it a good stir and enjoy your iron-boosting quinoa breakfast porridge!

This quinoa breakfast porridge combines the iron-rich quinoa with dried apricots and almonds for added iron content. The mixed berries provide a vitamin C boost to enhance iron absorption. The warm and comforting porridge is a great way to start your day and support your iron deficiency anemia. As always, consult a healthcare professional or registered dietitian if you have specific dietary concerns or questions about managing your anemia.

Nutrient-Packed Lunch Ideas

Here are some nutrient-packed lunch ideas specifically designed to support iron deficiency anemia:

1. Spinach and Lentil Salad:
   - Fresh spinach leaves (iron source)
   - Cooked green or brown lentils (iron and protein)
   - Sliced strawberries or oranges (vitamin C)
   - Chopped almonds or pumpkin seeds (iron and zinc)
   - Feta cheese (calcium)
   - Dress with a vinaigrette made with lemon juice (vitamin C) and olive oil

2. Quinoa and Chickpea Buddha Bowl:

- Cooked quinoa (protein, fiber)
- Chickpeas (iron and protein)
- Steamed broccoli and kale (iron and fiber)
- Shredded carrots and red cabbage (antioxidants)
- Avocado slices (healthy fats)
- Drizzle with tahini dressing (iron and healthy fats)

3. Tofu and Vegetable Stir-Fry:

- Cubed tofu (protein, iron)
- Assorted stir-fry vegetables (bell peppers, bok choy, snap peas)
- Quinoa or brown rice (fiber, protein)
- Stir-fry sauce with ginger, garlic, and low-sodium soy sauce
- Sesame seeds (iron and zinc) for topping

4. Black Bean and Quinoa Burrito Bowl:

- Cooked quinoa (protein, fiber)
- Black beans (iron and protein)
- Sautéed bell peppers and onions (vitamin C)
- Sliced avocado (healthy fats)
- Salsa and lime juice (vitamin C) for flavor

5. Salmon and Spinach Wrap:
- Whole-grain tortilla wrap
- Baked or grilled salmon (iron and omega-3 fatty acids)
- Fresh spinach leaves (iron)
- Sliced bell peppers and cucumber (vitamin C)
- Greek yogurt-based dressing with dill and lemon zest

6. Iron-Rich Vegetable Soup:
- Lentils or beans (iron and protein)
- Spinach or kale (iron)

- Carrots, celery, and tomatoes (vitamins and minerals)
- Whole-grain roll or bread on the side

7. Nut Butter and Banana Sandwich:
- Whole-grain bread (fiber, iron)
- Nut butter (iron and healthy fats)
- Sliced banana (potassium)
- Chia seeds (iron and fiber) sprinkled on top

These lunch ideas incorporate iron-rich ingredients like spinach, lentils, chickpeas, and quinoa while ensuring you also have sources of vitamin C and other essential nutrients to support iron absorption. Remember to consult a healthcare professional or registered dietitian if you have specific dietary concerns related to your iron deficiency anemia.

Lentil and Chickpea Salad

Here's a delicious and nutrient-packed Lentil and Chickpea Salad recipe that provides a combination of iron-rich legumes along with other wholesome ingredients:

Lentil and Chickpea Salad:

Ingredients:

- 1 cup cooked green or brown lentils (iron and protein)
- 1 cup cooked chickpeas (iron and protein)
- 1 cup diced cucumber
- 1 cup diced bell peppers (assorted colors for added vitamins)
- 1/2 cup diced red onion
- 1/4 cup chopped fresh parsley (flavor and nutrients)

- 1/4 cup crumbled feta cheese (calcium)
- 1/4 cup chopped almonds or pumpkin seeds (iron and crunch)
- Juice of 1 lemon (vitamin C)
- 2 tablespoons extra-virgin olive oil
- Salt and pepper to taste

Instructions:

- In a large bowl, combine the cooked lentils, cooked chickpeas, diced cucumber, diced bell peppers, diced red onion, and chopped parsley.
- In a small bowl, whisk together the lemon juice, extra-virgin olive oil, salt, and pepper to create the dressing.
- Pour the dressing over the salad and toss everything together until well combined.

- Gently fold in the crumbled feta cheese and chopped almonds or pumpkin seeds.
- Taste and adjust seasonings as needed.
- Serve the lentil and chickpea salad as a hearty and nutritious lunch option.

This Lentil and Chickpea Salad is not only rich in iron and protein but also packed with a variety of colorful vegetables and other nutrient-dense ingredients. The lemon juice in the dressing provides a dose of vitamin C to enhance iron absorption. It's a satisfying and well-balanced meal that can help support your iron deficiency anemia. As always, consult a healthcare professional or registered dietitian if you have specific dietary concerns or questions about managing your anemia.

Turkey and Spinach Wrap

Here's a tasty and nutrient-packed Turkey and Spinach Wrap recipe that combines lean protein, iron-rich greens, and other delicious ingredients:

Turkey and Spinach Wrap:

Ingredients:

- 1 whole-grain or whole-wheat tortilla wrap
- 4-6 slices of lean turkey breast (protein)
- Handful of fresh spinach leaves (iron)
- Sliced cucumbers and tomatoes (vitamins and crunch)
- Thinly sliced red onion (flavor)
- Hummus or Greek yogurt-based dressing (optional, for extra flavor)

- Salt, pepper, and your favorite herbs/spices

Instructions:

- Lay the tortilla wrap on a clean surface or plate.

- Layer the fresh spinach leaves evenly over the wrap.

- Arrange the slices of lean turkey breast on top of the spinach.

- Add sliced cucumbers, tomatoes, and red onion.

- If desired, spread a thin layer of hummus or drizzle a Greek yogurt-based dressing over the veggies for added flavor.

- Season with a pinch of salt, pepper, and your choice of herbs or spices.

- Carefully fold in the sides of the wrap, then roll it up tightly from the bottom to create your wrap.
- Slice the wrap in half diagonally, if preferred.
- Serve your Turkey and Spinach Wrap with a side of fresh fruit or a small salad.

This Turkey and Spinach Wrap is a balanced and nutritious option that provides protein from the turkey, iron from the spinach, and a variety of vitamins and minerals from the veggies. You can customize the wrap by adding other ingredients like avocado, grated carrots, or a sprinkle of feta cheese. Enjoy this satisfying and healthful lunch! If you have any specific dietary concerns, consulting a healthcare professional or

registered dietitian can provide personalized
guidance.

Tofu and Vegetable Stir-Fry

Here's a delicious and nutrient-packed Tofu and Vegetable Stir-Fry recipe that combines protein-rich tofu with a variety of colorful vegetables:

Tofu and Vegetable Stir-Fry:

Ingredients:

- 1 block of firm tofu, pressed and cubed (protein)
- Assorted vegetables (bell peppers, broccoli, carrots, snap peas, etc.)
- 1 tablespoon sesame oil or cooking oil
- 2 cloves garlic, minced
- 1 tablespoon grated ginger
- Low-sodium soy sauce or tamari, to taste

- 1 tablespoon cornstarch mixed with 2 tablespoons water (for sauce thickening)
- Optional toppings: sesame seeds, chopped green onions

Instructions:

- In a large pan or wok, heat the sesame oil over medium-high heat.
- Add the cubed tofu and stir-fry until it's lightly browned on all sides. Remove tofu from the pan and set aside.
- In the same pan, add a bit more oil if needed and sauté the minced garlic and grated ginger for about 1 minute until fragrant.
- Add the assorted vegetables to the pan and stir-fry until they're slightly tender yet still crisp.

- Push the vegetables to the side of the pan and add the cooked tofu back to the center.

- In a small bowl, mix the cornstarch and water to create a sauce thickener.

- Pour the cornstarch mixture and a drizzle of low-sodium soy sauce over the tofu and vegetables. Toss everything together to coat evenly.

- Continue stir-frying for another minute until the sauce thickens and coats the tofu and vegetables.

- Taste and adjust the seasoning with more soy sauce if needed.

- Remove from heat and serve your Tofu and Vegetable Stir-Fry over cooked quinoa or brown rice.

- Garnish with sesame seeds and chopped green onions, if desired.

This Tofu and Vegetable Stir-Fry is not only packed with protein from the tofu but also provides an array of vitamins, minerals, and fiber from the colorful vegetables. The combination of flavors and textures makes for a satisfying and nutritious meal. Feel free to customize the vegetables and sauce to your preference. As always, consulting a healthcare professional or registered dietitian can provide personalized guidance based on your dietary needs and goals.

Wholesome Dinner Dishes

Here are some wholesome and iron-rich dinner dish ideas specifically tailored to support individuals with iron deficiency anemia:

1. **Beef and Broccoli Stir-Fry:**
   - Lean beef strips (iron and protein)
   - Broccoli florets (iron and fiber)
   - Sliced bell peppers and carrots (vitamin C)
   - Low-sodium soy sauce or tamari
   - Serve with brown rice or quinoa
2. **Lentil and Vegetable Stew:**
   - Red or green lentils (iron and protein)
   - Assorted vegetables (spinach, carrots, tomatoes, etc.)
   - Vegetable broth

- Herbs and spices for flavor
- Serve with whole-grain bread or roll

3. Spinach and Chickpea Curry:

- Chickpeas (iron and protein)
- Fresh spinach (iron)
- Coconut milk (healthy fats)
- Curry spices (turmeric, cumin, coriander, etc.)
- Serve with brown rice or whole-grain naan

4. Turkey and Spinach Meatballs with Tomato Sauce:

- Ground turkey (iron and protein)
- Chopped spinach (iron)
- Whole-grain breadcrumbs
- Tomato sauce (vitamin C)
- Whole-grain pasta or zucchini noodles

5. Iron-Rich Veggie Stir-Fry:

- Tofu cubes (iron and protein)

- Spinach (iron)
- Assorted stir-fry vegetables (bell peppers, snap peas, etc.)
- Brown rice or quinoa
- Stir-fry sauce with garlic, ginger, and low-sodium soy sauce

6. **Quinoa and Black Bean Bowl:**
   - Cooked quinoa (protein, iron, and fiber)
   - Black beans (iron and protein)
   - Sautéed kale or collard greens (iron)
   - Sliced avocado (healthy fats)
   - Drizzle with lemon juice and olive oil

7. **Salmon and Sweet Potato Hash:**
   - Baked or grilled salmon (omega-3 fatty acids, protein)
   - Cubed roasted sweet potatoes (iron)
   - Sautéed spinach or kale (iron)

- Top with a poached egg for extra protein

Remember to pair iron-rich foods with sources of vitamin C (such as bell peppers, citrus fruits, and tomatoes) to enhance iron absorption. These wholesome dinner dishes provide a balance of nutrients while focusing on iron-rich ingredients to help support iron deficiency anemia. As always, consult a healthcare professional or registered dietitian for personalized guidance based on your individual dietary needs.

Beef and Broccoli Stir-Fry

Here's a delicious Beef and Broccoli Stir-Fry recipe that provides a flavorful and iron-rich meal:

Beef and Broccoli Stir-Fry:
Ingredients:

- 1/2 pound lean beef (sirloin or flank steak), thinly sliced (iron and protein)
- 2 cups broccoli florets (iron and fiber)
- 1 red bell pepper, sliced (vitamin C)
- 2 cloves garlic, minced
- 1 teaspoon fresh ginger, minced
- 2 tablespoons low-sodium soy sauce or tamari
- 1 tablespoon oyster sauce (optional)
- 1 teaspoon sesame oil

- 1 tablespoon cornstarch mixed with 2 tablespoons water (for sauce thickening)

- 2 tablespoons cooking oil (canola, peanut, or sesame oil)

- Sesame seeds for garnish (optional)

- Cooked brown rice or quinoa for serving

Instructions:

- In a bowl, combine the sliced beef with minced garlic, minced ginger, and 1 tablespoon of soy sauce. Allow it to marinate while you prepare the other ingredients.

- In a small bowl, mix the cornstarch with water to create a sauce thickener.

- Heat a wok or large skillet over high heat. Add 1 tablespoon of cooking oil and swirl to coat the pan.

- Add the marinated beef to the pan and stir-fry until it's cooked to your desired doneness. Remove the beef from the pan and set it aside.

- In the same pan, add another tablespoon of cooking oil. Add the broccoli florets and stir-fry for a couple of minutes until they start to turn bright green.

- Add the sliced red bell pepper and continue to stir-fry for another minute.

- Push the vegetables to the side of the pan and pour the cornstarch mixture into the center. Stir quickly to thicken.

- Return the cooked beef to the pan and toss everything together.

- Drizzle the remaining tablespoon of soy sauce and sesame oil over the stir-fry. If using oyster sauce, add it now as well.

- Stir-fry for another minute to combine all the flavors and ensure the beef and vegetables are well coated.

- Remove from heat and serve your Beef and Broccoli Stir-Fry over cooked brown rice or quinoa.

- Garnish with sesame seeds, if desired.

-

This Beef and Broccoli Stir-Fry is a delightful combination of iron-rich beef and broccoli, with the addition of vitamin C from the red bell pepper. It's a well-balanced and flavorful dish that can help support iron deficiency anemia. Enjoy it as a delicious and nutritious dinner option! As always, if you have specific dietary concerns or questions, consulting a healthcare professional or registered dietitian is recommended.

Salmon with Quinoa and Asparagus

Ingredients:

- 2 salmon fillets (omega-3 fatty acids, protein)
- 1 cup quinoa, rinsed (protein, fiber)
- 2 cups asparagus spears, trimmed (iron and fiber)
- 2 tablespoons olive oil
- Lemon zest and juice (vitamin C)
- Fresh dill or other herbs for garnish
- Salt and pepper to taste

Instructions:

- Preheat your oven to 375°F (190°C).
- Place the salmon fillets on a baking sheet lined with parchment paper. Drizzle with a bit of olive oil and season with salt and pepper.

- Bake the salmon in the preheated oven for about 12-15 minutes or until it flakes easily with a fork.

- While the salmon is baking, prepare the quinoa according to the package instructions.

- In a separate pan, heat the remaining olive oil over medium heat. Add the trimmed asparagus spears and sauté for about 4-5 minutes until they are tender but still slightly crisp.

- Once the quinoa is cooked, fluff it with a fork and season with lemon zest and a squeeze of lemon juice.

- To serve, divide the cooked quinoa among plates, top with baked salmon fillets, and arrange the sautéed asparagus on the side.

- Garnish with fresh dill or other herbs of your choice.

This Salmon with Quinoa and Asparagus dish provides a combination of protein from the salmon and quinoa, iron from the asparagus, and a burst of vitamin C from the lemon. It's a flavorful and wholesome dinner option that offers a variety of nutrients. Enjoy this nutritious and satisfying meal! If you have specific dietary concerns or questions, consulting a healthcare professional or registered dietitian is recommended.

Black Bean and Sweet Potato Chili

Ingredients:

- 2 cups cooked black beans (iron and protein)
- 2 medium sweet potatoes, peeled and diced (iron and fiber)
- 1 onion, chopped
- 3 cloves garlic, minced
- 1 red bell pepper, diced (vitamin C)
- 1 can (14 oz) diced tomatoes (vitamin C)
- 1 cup vegetable broth
- 1 tablespoon chili powder
- 1 teaspoon ground cumin
- 1 teaspoon paprika
- 1/2 teaspoon ground cinnamon
- Salt and pepper to taste
- 2 tablespoons olive oil

- Optional toppings: chopped fresh cilantro, shredded cheese, Greek yogurt

Instructions:

- In a large pot, heat the olive oil over medium heat. Add the chopped onion and sauté until translucent.

- Add the minced garlic, diced sweet potatoes, and red bell pepper. Sauté for a few minutes until the vegetables start to soften.

- Stir in the chili powder, ground cumin, paprika, and ground cinnamon. Cook for another minute until the spices are fragrant.

- Add the cooked black beans, diced tomatoes (with their juices), and vegetable broth to the pot. Stir to combine.

- Bring the chili to a simmer, then reduce the heat to low. Cover and let it cook for about 20-25 minutes, or until the sweet potatoes are tender.
- Season with salt and pepper to taste.
- Serve your Black Bean and Sweet Potato Chili in bowls, topped with optional toppings like chopped fresh cilantro, shredded cheese, or a dollop of Greek yogurt.

This Black Bean and Sweet Potato Chili is not only rich in iron from the black beans and sweet potatoes but also provides a variety of flavors and textures. The combination of spices and the addition of vitamin C-rich red bell pepper and diced tomatoes help enhance iron absorption. It's a hearty and nourishing dinner option that can be enjoyed on its own or with a side of whole-grain bread. As always, consulting a healthcare professional or registered dietitian for personalized guidance is recommended.

Snacks and Sides for Sustained Energy

Here are some nutrient-rich snacks and sides that can provide sustained energy and support individuals with iron deficiency anemia:

Snacks:

- Trail Mix: Create a mix of nuts (such as almonds, walnuts, and cashews) and dried fruits (raisins, apricots) for a balanced snack that combines healthy fats, protein, and iron-rich foods.

- Greek Yogurt Parfait: Layer Greek yogurt (protein and calcium) with fresh berries (vitamin C), chopped nuts (iron and protein), and a drizzle of honey for sweetness.

- Apple Slices with Nut Butter: Dip apple slices (fiber and vitamin C) into almond or peanut butter (iron and healthy fats) for a satisfying and nutrient-packed snack.

- Hummus and Veggie Sticks: Pair hummus (protein and iron) with carrot, celery, and bell pepper sticks (vitamin C) for a crunchy and iron-boosting snack.

- Oatmeal with Berries: A bowl of oatmeal (fiber and iron) topped with fresh berries (vitamin C) and a sprinkle of chia seeds (iron and fiber) makes for a nourishing snack.

Sides:

- Quinoa Salad: Prepare a quinoa salad with chopped vegetables (bell peppers, cucumbers, tomatoes) and beans (iron and protein), dressed with lemon juice (vitamin C) and olive oil.
- Spinach Salad: Create a spinach salad with baby spinach leaves (iron) and top it with grilled chicken or tofu (protein), sliced strawberries (vitamin C), and a light vinaigrette.
- Roasted Brussels Sprouts: Roast Brussels sprouts (iron and fiber) with a drizzle of olive oil and a sprinkle of Parmesan cheese (calcium) for a delicious side dish.
- Steamed Broccoli with Almonds: Steam broccoli florets (iron) and toss

them with sliced almonds (iron and healthy fats) for an iron-rich and crunchy side.

- Brown Rice Pilaf: Prepare a brown rice pilaf with sautéed onions, garlic, and chopped nuts (iron), and mix in dried cranberries (vitamin C) for a flavorful side.

These snacks and sides provide a combination of iron-rich foods along with other nutrients to help support sustained energy and manage iron deficiency anemia. Incorporating a variety of foods and flavors into your diet can contribute to a well-balanced and nourishing eating plan. As always, consulting a healthcare professional or registered dietitian for personalized guidance is recommended.

Roasted Chickpea Snack

Roasted chickpeas make for a delicious and crunchy snack that's also packed with protein and iron. Here's how to make Roasted Chickpea Snacks:

Roasted Chickpea Snack:

Ingredients:

- 1 can (15 oz) chickpeas (garbanzo beans), drained and rinsed
- 1-2 tablespoons olive oil
- Seasonings of your choice (such as chili powder, cumin, paprika, garlic powder, onion powder, cayenne pepper, or a blend)
- Salt and pepper to taste

Instructions:

- Preheat your oven to 400°F (200°C).

- Pat the rinsed chickpeas dry with a paper towel. This step helps them get crispy during roasting.

- In a bowl, toss the chickpeas with olive oil until they are evenly coated.

- Add your choice of seasonings, salt, and pepper to the chickpeas. Mix well to ensure they are coated with the flavors.

- Spread the seasoned chickpeas in a single layer on a baking sheet lined with parchment paper.

- Roast the chickpeas in the preheated oven for about 25-30 minutes, or until they are golden brown and crispy. Shake the baking sheet occasionally to ensure even roasting.

- Remove from the oven and let the chickpeas cool slightly before enjoying.

Roasted chickpeas are a wonderful iron-rich snack option that also provides a satisfying crunch. You can customize the seasonings to your taste, whether you prefer a savory, spicy, or even a slightly sweet flavor. Make a big batch and store them in an airtight container for convenient snacking.

Remember to pair these with a vitamin C-rich option like sliced bell peppers or citrus fruits to enhance iron absorption. As always, consulting a healthcare professional or registered dietitian for personalized guidance is recommended.

Hummus and Veggie Platter

Hummus and Veggie Platter is a fantastic and nutritious option, especially for individuals with iron deficiency anemia. Here's how you can create a satisfying and iron-rich hummus and veggie platter:

Hummus and Veggie Platter:
Ingredients:

- Hummus (store-bought or homemade) – chickpeas are an excellent source of iron
- Assorted fresh vegetables (choose a variety of colors for different nutrients):
- Carrot sticks (iron)
- Bell pepper strips (vitamin C)

- Cucumber slices
- Cherry tomatoes (vitamin C)

Celery sticks

- Broccoli florets (iron)
- Cauliflower florets
- Whole-grain pita bread or whole-grain crackers (fiber and complex carbs)
- Optional garnishes: drizzle of olive oil, chopped fresh herbs, olives

Instructions:

- Prepare the vegetables: Wash, peel, and chop the vegetables into bite-sized pieces or sticks.
- Arrange the vegetables on a large platter or serving tray, creating a colorful and inviting display.
- Place a bowl of hummus in the center of the platter.

- If using pita bread, cut it into triangles or squares and arrange them around the hummus.
- Add whole-grain crackers to the platter for additional crunch and fiber.
- Drizzle a bit of olive oil over the hummus for extra flavor, if desired.
- Garnish with chopped fresh herbs or olives for a finishing touch.

To enjoy, simply dip the assorted veggies and whole-grain pita or crackers into the hummus. The combination of iron-rich chickpeas in the hummus and vitamin C-rich vegetables creates a great balance for enhancing iron absorption. This platter is not only delicious but also visually appealing, making it perfect for gatherings or a wholesome snack at home. As always, consulting a healthcare professional or registered dietitian for personalized guidance is recommended.

Iron-Rich Trail Mix

Ingredients:

- Almonds (iron and healthy fats)
- Pumpkin seeds (iron and zinc)
- Dried apricots (iron and vitamin C)
- Raisins or dried cranberries (iron and vitamin C)
- Dark chocolate chunks (iron)
- Whole-grain cereal or granola (iron and fiber)
- Optional: cashews (iron), walnuts (iron), dried figs (iron and fiber)

Instructions:

- In a bowl, combine equal parts of almonds, pumpkin seeds, dried apricots, raisins or dried cranberries,

dark   chocolate   chunks,   and
whole-grain cereal or granola.

- Feel free to add a handful of cashews,
  walnuts, and dried figs if you like.
- Mix everything together until well
  combined.

Portion the trail mix into small resealable bags or containers for easy grab-and-go snacking. The combination of iron-rich nuts and seeds with dried fruits high in vitamin C makes this trail mix a great choice for boosting iron absorption. It's a convenient and tasty snack to enjoy on the go or whenever you need an energy boost. As always, consulting a healthcare professional or registered dietitian for personalized guidance is recommended, especially if you have specific dietary needs or concerns.

Sweet Treats for Anemia Support

Here are some sweet treat ideas that not only satisfy your taste buds but also provide a dose of iron or enhance iron absorption:

1. Dark Chocolate-Covered Strawberries:
Dip fresh strawberries (vitamin C) in melted dark chocolate (iron) for a delicious and antioxidant-rich treat.

2. Iron-Boosting Smoothie Popsicles:
Blend together iron-rich ingredients like spinach, strawberries (vitamin C), Greek yogurt (calcium), and a touch of honey. Pour into popsicle molds and freeze for a refreshing treat.

3. Chocolate-Dipped Bananas:

Slice bananas and dip them in melted dark chocolate. For an extra boost, sprinkle some crushed almonds (iron) before the chocolate hardens.

4. Chia Seed Pudding:

Make chia seed pudding with almond milk (iron), chia seeds (iron and fiber), and a touch of honey. Top with berries (vitamin C) for added flavor and nutrients.

5. Yogurt Parfait with Iron-Rich Toppings:

Layer Greek yogurt (protein and calcium) with chopped dates (iron), dried apricots (iron and vitamin C), and a sprinkle of crushed nuts (iron) for crunch.

6. Iron-Enhanced Fruit Salad:

Combine iron-rich fruits like watermelon, pomegranate seeds, and kiwi with a squeeze of lemon juice (vitamin C) for an extra boost.

7. Oatmeal Raisin Cookies:
Bake oatmeal cookies with whole-grain oats (iron and fiber) and raisins (iron). Use honey or maple syrup as a natural sweetener.

8. Iron-Rich Nut Butter Energy Balls:
Mix nut butter (iron and healthy fats), chopped dates (iron), rolled oats, and a sprinkle of chia seeds. Shape into small energy balls and refrigerate.

Remember, while enjoying these sweet treats, it's a good idea to combine them with sources of vitamin C (like fruits) to enhance iron absorption. Moderation is key, and consulting a healthcare professional or registered dietitian for personalized guidance is recommended, especially if you have specific dietary concerns or conditions.

Dark Chocolate Nut Bites

Ingredients:

- Dark chocolate (70% cocoa or higher) - chopped or chocolate chips (iron)
- Assorted nuts (choose from almonds, walnuts, cashews, pistachios, etc.) - chopped or whole (iron and healthy fats)
- Optional: dried cranberries or cherries (iron and vitamin C), shredded coconut, sea salt flakes

Instructions:
- Melt the dark chocolate in a microwave-safe bowl or using a double boiler.

- Line a mini muffin tin or a baking sheet with parchment paper or mini muffin liners.

- Spoon a small amount of melted chocolate into each mini muffin cup or liner, just enough to cover the bottom.

- Place a few pieces of assorted nuts into each cup on top of the chocolate. You can use a combination of nuts or stick to your favorite variety.

- If desired, add a few dried cranberries or cherries for a touch of sweetness and vitamin C.

- Spoon more melted chocolate over the nuts and dried fruit to cover them completely.

- If using, sprinkle a pinch of shredded coconut or a few sea salt flakes on top of each bite for added flavor and texture.

- Place the muffin tin or baking sheet in the refrigerator to allow the chocolate to set. This will take about 30 minutes to an hour.

- Once the chocolate is fully set, carefully remove the Dark Chocolate Nut Bites from the muffin tin or peel away the muffin liners.

Enjoy these Dark Chocolate Nut Bites as a delightful and iron-rich sweet treat. The combination of dark chocolate and nuts provides a satisfying balance of flavors and textures, making it a perfect bite-sized snack. Remember to pair this treat with a source of vitamin C (such as a piece of citrus fruit) to enhance iron absorption. As always, consult a healthcare professional or registered dietitian for personalized guidance, especially if you have specific dietary needs or concerns.

Berry and Spinach Smoothie

Ingredients:

- 1 cup mixed berries (such as strawberries, blueberries, and raspberries) - rich in antioxidants and vitamin C
- 1 cup fresh spinach leaves - a source of iron and other essential nutrients
- 1 ripe banana - natural sweetness and potassium
- 1/2 cup Greek yogurt - protein and probiotics
- 1 tablespoon chia seeds or flax seeds - omega-3 fatty acids and fiber
- 1 cup unsweetened almond milk or your preferred milk choice

- Optional: honey or maple syrup for added sweetness, ice cubes for a chilled texture

Instructions:

- Place the mixed berries, fresh spinach, ripe banana, Greek yogurt, chia seeds (or flax seeds), and unsweetened almond milk in a blender.
- If desired, add a drizzle of honey or maple syrup for extra sweetness.
- Blend on high speed until all the ingredients are well combined and the smoothie is smooth and creamy.
- If you prefer a thicker smoothie, you can add a handful of ice cubes and blend again until the desired consistency is reached.

- Taste the smoothie and adjust sweetness if needed by adding a bit more honey or maple syrup.
- Pour the Berry and Spinach Smoothie into glasses and enjoy immediately.

This Berry and Spinach Smoothie is not only refreshing and delicious but also provides a good amount of iron from the spinach, antioxidants from the berries, and a variety of other essential nutrients. It's a great way to sneak in some greens and fruits into your diet, especially for individuals with iron deficiency anemia. As always, consulting a healthcare professional or registered dietitian for personalized guidance is recommended, especially if you have specific dietary needs or concerns.

Iron-Enriched Dessert Options

Here are some iron-enriched dessert options that can satisfy your sweet tooth while providing a boost of iron:

1. Dark Chocolate-Dipped Strawberries:
Dip fresh strawberries (vitamin C) into melted dark chocolate (iron) for a delicious and antioxidant-rich treat.

2. Iron-Rich Fruit Parfait:
Layer Greek yogurt (protein and calcium) with chopped dried apricots (iron and vitamin C), sliced bananas, and a sprinkle of chopped nuts (iron) for crunch.

3. Chocolate-Banana Smoothie Bowl:

Blend together ripe bananas (iron and potassium), cocoa powder (iron), and Greek yogurt for a creamy and iron-rich smoothie bowl. Top with granola (iron and fiber) and sliced almonds (iron).

4. Black Bean Brownies:
Replace some or all of the flour in your favorite brownie recipe with pureed black beans (iron and protein) for a nutrient-packed dessert.

5. Iron-Enhanced Oat Cookies:
Bake oat cookies with rolled oats (iron and fiber) and dried cherries (iron and vitamin C) or raisins. You can also add chopped nuts for an extra iron boost.

6. Iron-Infused Chia Seed Pudding:

Make chia seed pudding using almond milk (iron), chia seeds (iron and fiber), and a touch of cocoa powder for a chocolatey twist.

7. Quinoa Pudding:
Cook quinoa (iron and protein) with milk and sweetener of your choice until creamy. Add vanilla extract and a sprinkle of cinnamon for flavor.

8. Iron-Enriched Energy Balls:
Combine dates (iron), almond butter (iron and healthy fats), rolled oats (iron and fiber), and a bit of cocoa powder to create nutrient-dense energy balls.

Remember, while enjoying these iron-enriched desserts, consider pairing them with vitamin C-rich foods like citrus fruits, berries, or bell peppers to enhance iron absorption. Moderation is key, and consulting a healthcare professional or registered dietitian for personalized guidance is recommended, especially if you have specific dietary concerns or conditions.

Lifestyle Tips to Enhance Iron Absorption

Here are some lifestyle tips to help enhance iron absorption and support individuals with iron deficiency anemia:

1. Consume Iron-Rich Foods: Incorporate a variety of iron-rich foods into your diet, such as lean meats, poultry, fish, beans, lentils, tofu, nuts, seeds, dark leafy greens, and whole grains.

2. Pair with Vitamin C: Include foods high in vitamin C, like citrus fruits, strawberries, bell peppers, and tomatoes, with iron-rich foods to enhance iron absorption.

3. Avoid Calcium Interference: Avoid consuming calcium-rich foods and supplements at the same time as iron-rich foods, as calcium can inhibit iron absorption. Aim to separate them by a few hours.

4. Choose Cooking Methods Wisely: Opt for cooking methods that preserve iron content, such as steaming or sautéing. Cast iron cookware can also increase iron content in cooked foods.

5. Limit Coffee and Tea: Avoid drinking coffee or tea with meals, as they contain compounds that can hinder iron absorption. If you do consume them, try waiting at least an hour after eating.

6. Consider Vitamin A: Include foods rich in vitamin A, like sweet potatoes, carrots, and dark leafy greens, as vitamin A supports iron metabolism.

7. Manage Stress: High stress levels can affect digestion and nutrient absorption. Incorporate relaxation techniques like meditation, deep breathing, or yoga to help manage stress.

8. Stay Hydrated: Drink plenty of water throughout the day to support overall digestion and absorption of nutrients.

9. Monitor Medications: Some medications can affect iron absorption. Consult your healthcare provider to discuss any potential interactions or adjustments.

10. Regular Blood Tests: Schedule regular follow-up appointments with your healthcare provider for blood tests to monitor your iron levels and adjust your diet or treatment plan as needed.

11. Balanced Diet: Maintain a balanced diet that includes a variety of nutrients to support overall health and well-being.

12. Work with a Professional: Consult a registered dietitian or healthcare professional to develop a personalized plan that addresses your specific iron deficiency anemia needs.

Remember that everyone's iron needs are unique, and it's important to work with a healthcare professional to create a plan that suits your individual situation. These lifestyle tips, combined with a well-balanced diet and appropriate medical care, can help optimize iron absorption and support your overall health

Pairing Foods for Better Iron Uptake

Pairing foods strategically can enhance iron uptake and absorption. Here's how you can optimize your meals to improve iron absorption:

1. Iron-Rich Foods and Vitamin C Sources:
Pair iron-rich foods like beans, lentils, and spinach with vitamin C-rich sources such as citrus fruits, strawberries, bell peppers, and tomatoes. Vitamin C enhances non-heme iron absorption from plant-based sources.

2. Meat and Vitamin C:
If consuming animal-based iron sources like lean meats, poultry, or fish, include a side of

vegetables or fruits high in vitamin C to boost iron absorption.

3. Iron and Beta-Carotene:
Combine iron-rich foods with those containing beta-carotene, like sweet potatoes, carrots, and dark leafy greens. Beta-carotene supports iron absorption and metabolism.

4. Heme Iron and Non-Heme Iron:
Combine heme iron sources (found in animal products) with non-heme iron sources (found in plant-based foods) to optimize absorption. For instance, have lean meat with a side of spinach salad.

5. Iron and Fiber:

Include foods rich in both iron and dietary fiber, such as lentils, quinoa, and whole grains. Fiber can promote healthy digestion, which supports iron absorption.

6. Calcium and Iron:
While calcium can inhibit iron absorption, consuming small amounts of calcium-rich foods like yogurt or cheese with iron-rich meals won't significantly impact absorption. Just avoid consuming large calcium doses at the same time as iron-rich foods.

7. Avoid Inhibitors:
Limit or avoid foods high in inhibitors like phytates (found in grains) and polyphenols (found in tea and coffee) during iron-rich meals, as they can hinder iron absorption.

8. Iron-Fortified Foods with Vitamin C:

If consuming iron-fortified foods (like cereals), pair them with a vitamin C source to improve iron uptake.

Remember, a balanced and varied diet plays a key role in maintaining good health. Consult with a healthcare professional or registered dietitian for personalized guidance, especially if you have specific dietary concerns or medical conditions. They can help create a meal plan that optimizes iron absorption based on your individual needs.

Cooking Techniques to Preserve Iron Content

Here are some cooking techniques that can help preserve the iron content in your food and improve its availability for absorption:

1. Steaming: Steaming is a gentle cooking method that helps retain the iron content of vegetables. Steam your vegetables until they are tender but still vibrant in color.

2. Sautéing: Sautéing quickly over high heat with a small amount of oil can help preserve iron in vegetables while enhancing their flavor and texture.

3. Blanching: Briefly blanching vegetables in boiling water before cooking can help

preserve their iron content. This method is particularly useful for greens like spinach and kale.

4. Quick Cooking: Cooking foods for a shorter duration can help maintain their iron content. Avoid overcooking vegetables to prevent excessive iron loss.

5. Using Cast Iron Cookware: Cooking with cast iron pots and pans can slightly increase the iron content of the food, especially when cooking acidic foods like tomatoes.

6. Acidic Ingredients: Cooking foods with acidic ingredients like tomatoes, citrus juice, or vinegar can help enhance the availability of non-heme iron from plant-based sources.

7. Avoid Excessive Heat: High temperatures and prolonged cooking times can lead to iron loss. Use moderate heat and cook foods for shorter durations whenever possible.

8. Combining Foods: Combining iron-rich foods with vitamin C-rich foods can enhance iron absorption. For example, add lemon juice to vegetables or meat dishes containing iron.

9. Minimize Water Usage: Cooking methods that use minimal water, such as steaming or stir-frying, can help reduce the leaching of iron into cooking water.

10. Soaking and Sprouting: Soaking and sprouting grains, legumes, and seeds can

help reduce phytates, which can inhibit iron absorption.

11. Resting Before Cutting: Allowing meat to rest for a few minutes after cooking before cutting helps retain more of its juices and iron content.

Remember that balanced and diverse meals, along with proper cooking techniques, contribute to a diet that supports iron absorption and overall nutritional needs. Consulting a registered dietitian or healthcare professional can provide personalized guidance on cooking and meal planning to optimize your iron intake.

Managing Iron Intake with Other Nutrients

Managing iron intake along with other nutrients is crucial for overall health. Here's how you can balance iron with other nutrients:

1. Vitamin C: Pair iron-rich foods with sources of vitamin C, like citrus fruits, bell peppers, and strawberries. Vitamin C enhances the absorption of non-heme iron from plant-based sources.

2. Calcium: While calcium can inhibit non-heme iron absorption, consuming small amounts of calcium-rich foods with iron-rich meals is generally fine. Avoid

consuming large calcium doses at the same time as iron-rich foods.

3. Fiber: Fiber is important for digestion, but consuming excessive fiber with iron-rich foods may hinder absorption. Aim for a balance between iron-rich foods and dietary fiber sources.

4. Phytates and Oxalates: Foods high in phytates (found in grains and legumes) and oxalates (found in spinach, beet greens, and nuts) can inhibit iron absorption. Soaking, sprouting, and cooking can help reduce their impact.

5. Zinc: Excessive zinc intake may interfere with iron absorption. If taking zinc

supplements, consider spacing them out from iron-rich meals.

6. Coffee and Tea: Tannins in coffee and tea can inhibit iron absorption. Avoid drinking them with iron-rich meals or consume them between meals.

7. Dairy and Iron-Rich Foods: Avoid consuming dairy products at the same time as iron-rich foods, as calcium can hinder iron absorption. Opt for separate consumption or small amounts with iron-rich meals.

8. Balanced Diet: Maintain a balanced diet that includes a variety of nutrients from different food groups to ensure overall health and prevent nutrient imbalances.

9. Moderation: While managing nutrient interactions is important, it's essential to focus on a well-rounded diet rather than overly restricting certain nutrients.

10. Individual Needs: Consider consulting a registered dietitian or healthcare professional to personalize your diet based on your unique nutritional needs and any underlying health conditions.

Remember, the goal is to create a balanced and diverse diet that meets your nutritional needs while optimizing iron absorption. Pay attention to the timing of certain foods and consult a healthcare professional for personalized guidance, especially if you have specific dietary concerns or medical conditions.

Meal Planning and Grocery Shopping for Anemia

Creating a well-balanced meal plan and making thoughtful choices during grocery shopping can help manage anemia and support optimal iron intake. Here's a step-by-step guide:

1. Assess Your Needs:

Determine your iron needs based on factors like age, gender, activity level, and any medical conditions.

Consult a healthcare professional or registered dietitian for personalized recommendations.

2. Plan Balanced Meals:

Include a variety of iron-rich foods such as lean meats, poultry, fish, beans, lentils, tofu, nuts, seeds, dark leafy greens, and whole grains.
Pair iron-rich foods with sources of vitamin C to enhance iron absorption.

3. Create a Weekly Meal Plan:
Plan your meals for the week, considering breakfast, lunch, dinner, and snacks.
Ensure each meal includes a balance of protein, carbohydrates, healthy fats, and a variety of nutrients.

4. Make a Grocery List:
Based on your meal plan, create a detailed grocery list of the ingredients you need.
Include iron-rich foods, sources of vitamin C, and other essential nutrients.

5. Grocery Shopping Tips:

Stick to the perimeter of the grocery store, where fresh produce, lean proteins, and whole grains are typically located.

Read labels to choose fortified foods and check for iron content.

Choose whole, minimally processed foods whenever possible.

6. Include Iron-Rich Foods:

Select a variety of iron-rich foods, such as lean meats (chicken, turkey, beef), fish, legumes (beans, lentils), tofu, nuts, seeds, and dark leafy greens (spinach, kale).

7. Opt for Vitamin C Sources:

Add vitamin C-rich foods to your cart, like citrus fruits (oranges, lemons), berries, bell peppers, and tomatoes.

8. Whole Grains and Fiber:
Choose whole grains like quinoa, brown rice, whole wheat pasta, and whole grain bread to provide fiber and other nutrients.

9. Dairy and Calcium:
Include calcium-rich foods like low-fat dairy, fortified plant-based milk, and leafy greens. Consume them at separate times from iron-rich meals.

10. Meal Prep:
Prepare components of meals in advance, such as chopping vegetables, cooking grains,

and marinating proteins, to make meal preparation easier during the week.

11. Hydration:
Don't forget to include water in your grocery list to stay hydrated throughout the day.

Remember, individual needs vary, and it's important to tailor your meal plan and grocery shopping to your specific requirements. Consulting a registered dietitian or healthcare professional can provide personalized guidance to help you create a balanced and nutrient-rich eating plan that supports your anemia management.

Weekly Meal Plans

Here's a sample weekly meal plan that focuses on iron-rich foods and nutrient balance to support individuals with anemia. Remember to customize portion sizes and specific food choices based on your individual needs and preferences:

Day 1:

Breakfast: Spinach and Mushroom Omelette (eggs, spinach, mushrooms)

Lunch: Lentil and Chickpea Salad (lentils, chickpeas, mixed vegetables)

Snack: Greek yogurt with mixed berries

Dinner: Grilled Chicken Breast with Quinoa and Steamed Broccoli (chicken, quinoa, broccoli)

Day 2:

Breakfast: Iron-Boosting Smoothie Bowl (spinach, berries, chia seeds)

Lunch: Tofu and Vegetable Stir-Fry (tofu, assorted vegetables)

Snack: Handful of almonds and an orange

Dinner: Salmon with Brown Rice and Asparagus (salmon, brown rice, asparagus)

Day 3:

Breakfast: Whole Grain Toast with Avocado and Poached Egg (whole grain bread, avocado, egg)

Lunch: Mixed Greens Salad with Grilled Steak (steak, mixed greens, bell peppers)

Snack: Carrot sticks with hummus

Dinner: Black Bean and Sweet Potato Chili (black beans, sweet potatoes, tomatoes)

Day 4:

Breakfast: Berry and Spinach Smoothie (mixed berries, spinach, Greek yogurt)

Lunch: Turkey and Spinach Wrap (turkey, whole wheat wrap, spinach)

Snack: Cottage cheese with sliced strawberries

Dinner: Beef and Broccoli Stir-Fry with Brown Rice (beef, broccoli, brown rice)

Day 5:

Breakfast: Quinoa Breakfast Porridge with Almond Butter (quinoa, almond butter)

Lunch: Chickpea and Spinach Salad (chickpeas, spinach, tomatoes)

Snack: Apple slices with peanut butter

Dinner: Chicken and Vegetable Stew (chicken, mixed vegetables, herbs)

Day 6:

Breakfast: Greek Yogurt Parfait with Mixed Nuts (Greek yogurt, mixed nuts, dried fruits)

Lunch: Spinach and Feta Stuffed Bell Peppers (spinach, bell peppers, feta cheese)

Snack: Trail mix with dried fruits and pumpkin seeds

Dinner: Lentil Curry with Brown Rice (lentils, brown rice, vegetables)

Day 7:

Breakfast: Whole Grain Pancakes with Berries (whole grain pancakes, mixed berries)

Lunch: Quinoa and Black Bean Salad (quinoa, black beans, mixed vegetables)

Snack: Cottage cheese with pineapple chunks

Dinner: Grilled Portobello Mushrooms with Couscous (portobello mushrooms, couscous, herbs)

Remember to adjust portion sizes, include vitamin C-rich foods, and stay hydrated throughout the week. This sample meal plan provides a variety of iron-rich options while maintaining a balanced and nutrient-rich diet. Consulting a registered dietitian or healthcare professional can help you tailor the plan to your individual needs and ensure you're meeting your nutritional requirements.

Stocking Your Pantry with Iron-Rich Foods

Stocking your pantry with a variety of iron-rich foods is essential for managing anemia and maintaining a balanced diet. Here's a list of iron-rich foods to keep in your pantry:

Grains and Legumes:

- Whole grains (brown rice, quinoa, oats, whole wheat pasta)
- Lentils (green, red, brown)
- Chickpeas and other beans (black beans, kidney beans, pinto beans)
- Black-eyed peas
- Split peas

Nuts and Seeds:

- Almonds
- Pumpkin seeds
- Sunflower seeds
- Chia seeds
- Flaxseeds

Nut Butters:

- Peanut butter
- Almond butter
- Cashew butter

Cereals and Breads:

- Iron-fortified breakfast cereals
- Whole grain bread

Dried Fruits:

- Raisins
- Apricots
- Dates
- Prunes

Canned Foods:

- Canned tuna or salmon
- Canned beans (rinse well before use to reduce sodium content)

Cooking Staples:

- Olive oil (for sautéing and cooking)
- Herbs and spices (for flavor and added nutrients)

Other Pantry Items:

- Dark chocolate (70% cocoa or higher)
- Quinoa (rich in protein and iron)
- Canned tomatoes (for vitamin C-rich sauces)
- Whole wheat flour (for baking)

Tips for Pantry Organization:

- Label and Rotate: Mark the purchase date on items to help you use the oldest ones first. This reduces the chances of items going bad before you get a chance to use them.

- Visibility: Organize your pantry so that you can easily see and access your iron-rich foods. This encourages you to use them more often.
- Meal Planning: Plan meals around the ingredients you have in your pantry to ensure you're incorporating iron-rich foods into your diet regularly.
- Healthy Snacks: Keep nutritious snacks like nuts, seeds, and dried fruits on hand for quick and satisfying options.
- Variety: Aim for a diverse selection of iron-rich foods to prevent monotony and ensure you're getting a range of nutrients.

- Stay Stocked: Regularly check your pantry items and restock when needed to maintain a consistent supply of iron-rich foods.

Remember to incorporate these pantry items into your meals and snacks as part of a balanced diet. Consulting a registered dietitian or healthcare professional can provide personalized guidance on creating a pantry that meets your individual nutritional needs.

Reading Labels and Choosing Fortified Products

Reading labels and choosing fortified products can be beneficial for individuals managing anemia. Here's how to navigate labels and make informed choices:

1. Check the Nutrition Facts:
Look for the "Iron" content in the Nutrition Facts panel. It will indicate the amount of iron present in the product.
Keep in mind that the Daily Value (DV) for iron is typically 18 mg. Aim for products that contribute a significant portion of this value.

2. Look for Fortification:

Check the ingredient list for terms like "iron-fortified," "iron-enriched," or "added iron." This indicates that the product has been supplemented with iron.

3. Assess Serving Size:
Be mindful of the serving size listed on the label. Make sure to adjust the iron content according to the amount you'll actually consume.

4. Consider Absorption Factors:
If the product is fortified with non-heme iron (plant-based iron), pairing it with vitamin C-rich foods can enhance absorption.

5. Choose Whole Foods Whenever Possible:
While fortified products can be helpful, whole food sources of iron are often more nutrient-dense and come with other essential nutrients.

Examples of Fortified Products:
- Iron-fortified breakfast cereals
- Fortified plant-based milk (such as almond, soy, or oat milk)
- Fortified orange juice or other fruit juices
- Iron-fortified granola bars or energy bars
- Fortified nut butters

Tips for Making Choices:
Compare labels to choose products with higher iron content per serving.

Be mindful of added sugars, sodium, and other additives in fortified products.

Incorporate fortified products into your diet as part of a well-rounded meal plan.

Consult a Professional:

If you're unsure about which fortified products to choose, or if you have specific dietary concerns, consult a registered dietitian or healthcare professional for personalized guidance.

Remember that fortified products can be a convenient way to increase your iron intake, but they should be part of a balanced diet that includes a variety of nutrient-rich whole foods.

Frequently Asked Questions about Anemia and Diet

1.What is Anemia

Anemia is a condition characterized by a decrease in the number of red blood cells or a low hemoglobin level, which can lead to reduced oxygen-carrying capacity in the blood.

2. How can diet affect anemia?

Diet plays a crucial role in managing anemia by providing essential nutrients like iron, vitamin B12, and folate, which are necessary for red blood cell production.

3. What are the best food sources of iron?

Good sources of iron include lean meats, poultry, fish, legumes, lentils, tofu, nuts, seeds, whole grains, and dark leafy greens.

4. How can I enhance iron absorption from plant-based foods?

Pair iron-rich plant-based foods with vitamin C-rich sources, like citrus fruits, bell peppers, or strawberries, to enhance iron absorption.

5. What foods should I avoid to improve iron absorption?

Limit consumption of calcium-rich foods and beverages like dairy products and fortified foods when consuming iron-rich meals, as calcium can inhibit iron absorption.

6. Are there foods that hinder iron absorption?

Foods high in phytates (found in grains and legumes) and polyphenols (found in tea, coffee, and certain spices) can inhibit iron absorption. Cooking, soaking, and fermenting can help reduce their impact.

7. Can I get enough iron from a vegetarian or vegan diet?

Yes, a well-planned vegetarian or vegan diet can provide sufficient iron by including plant-based iron sources and optimizing absorption through dietary strategies.

8. Should I take iron supplements?

Iron supplements may be recommended by a healthcare professional if your iron levels are significantly low. However, it's important to consult a doctor before starting any supplementation.

9. How does vitamin B12 deficiency relate to anemia?

Vitamin B12 deficiency can lead to a type of anemia called megaloblastic anemia, which affects red blood cell production. Animal products and fortified foods are common sources of vitamin B12.

10. Can anemia be managed solely through diet?

In some cases, mild anemia can be managed through diet alone, especially by increasing iron-rich foods. However, more severe cases may require medical intervention and supplements.

11. How often should I get my iron levels checked?

It's advisable to have your iron levels checked regularly, especially if you have a history of anemia or related health conditions. Consult your healthcare provider for guidance.

12. Can I improve my energy levels through diet if I have anemia?

A balanced diet rich in iron and other essential nutrients can contribute to improved energy levels over time for individuals with anemia.

Remember, the information provided is a general guideline. If you have specific questions or concerns about anemia and your diet, it's best to consult a registered dietitian or healthcare professional for personalized advice based on your individual needs and medical history.

Addressing Concerns About Vegetarian or Vegan Diets

Addressing concerns about vegetarian or vegan diets in relation to anemia is important. Here are common concerns and how to address them:

1. Iron Deficiency:

Concern: Plant-based diets may lack sufficient iron.

Solution: Include iron-rich plant foods such as lentils, beans, tofu, nuts, seeds, fortified cereals, and dark leafy greens. Pair these with vitamin C sources to enhance absorption. Consider periodic blood tests to monitor iron levels.

2. Vitamin B12 Deficiency:

Concern: Vitamin B12 is mostly found in animal products, which may be lacking in vegetarian or vegan diets.

Solution: Consume fortified plant-based milk, cereals, and nutritional yeast. If needed, consider vitamin B12 supplements or fortified foods. Regularly check B12 levels and consult a healthcare professional.

3. Protein Intake:

Concern: Vegetarian or vegan diets may not provide enough protein.

Solution: Incorporate diverse protein sources like beans, lentils, tofu, tempeh, quinoa, nuts, and seeds. Combining different plant proteins throughout the day can ensure adequate intake.

4. Calcium and Dairy:

Concern: Dairy is a common calcium source in non-vegetarian diets.

Solution: Choose fortified plant-based milk (like almond or soy milk) and include calcium-rich plant foods like leafy greens, almonds, and fortified orange juice.

5. Omega-3 Fatty Acids:

Concern: Fish is a primary source of omega-3 fatty acids.

Solution: Include flaxseeds, chia seeds, walnuts, and omega-3 fortified foods. Consider an algae-based omega-3 supplement.

6. Vitamin D:

Concern: Limited sun exposure and lack of dairy may impact vitamin D levels.

Solution: Spend time outdoors for sunlight exposure. Choose fortified plant-based milk and consider a vitamin D supplement, especially if recommended by a healthcare professional.

7. Nutrient Absorption:
Concern: Plant compounds may affect nutrient absorption.
Solution: Soak, sprout, or ferment grains, legumes, and seeds to reduce phytates. Cooking can also enhance nutrient availability.

8. Variety and Balance:
Concern: Over-reliance on processed foods in plant-based diets.
Solution: Focus on whole, nutrient-dense foods. Incorporate a variety of fruits,

vegetables, whole grains, legumes, nuts, and seeds.

9. Individualized Planning:
Concern: Properly planning a vegetarian or vegan diet can be complex.
Solution: Consult a registered dietitian with expertise in plant-based nutrition. They can help create a well-balanced meal plan that meets your nutritional needs.

Remember, a well-planned vegetarian or vegan diet can be nutritionally adequate and provide health benefits, but proper planning and informed choices are essential. Regular health check-ups and consultations with healthcare professionals can help address any concerns and ensure optimal health.

Conclusion and Empowerment

In conclusion, managing anemia through a well-balanced diet is both achievable and empowering. By understanding the importance of key nutrients like iron, vitamin B12, and folate, and incorporating a variety of nutrient-rich foods into your meals, you can take meaningful steps towards improving your iron levels and overall health.

Empowerment lies in your ability to make informed choices. With the knowledge of iron-rich food sources, absorption-enhancing strategies, and the support of healthcare professionals or registered dietitians, you have the tools to take charge of your anemia management journey.

Remember, every meal is an opportunity to nourish your body and support your well-being. Building a diet rich in lean meats, poultry, fish, legumes, whole grains, nuts, seeds, and dark leafy greens can contribute to your iron intake and help combat anemia. Pairing iron-rich foods with vitamin C sources and making thoughtful cooking choices further enhances absorption.

As you embark on this path, take pride in your efforts to create meals that promote health and vitality. Regular check-ups and consultations will guide your progress, ensuring that you're on the right track. With commitment, knowledge, and the support of healthcare professionals, you have the ability to overcome anemia and embrace a lifestyle that fosters lasting well-being.

Empower yourself with the understanding that each choice you make brings you closer to optimal health. Your journey towards managing anemia through a balanced and nutrient-rich diet is a testament to your dedication to self-care and a vibrant future.